COMPLETE GUIDE TO CHOLECYSTITIS

Your Essential Manual For Understanding, Treating, Beating Gallbladder Inflammation, Symptoms, Treatments, Surgery, And Nutrition Explained

DEHART HAIRSTON

DISCLAIMER

This book's content is only intended for general informative purposes. At the time of writing, the author has taken every precaution to guarantee that the material is correct and current. Nevertheless, the author disclaims all explicit and implicit representations and guarantees about the availability, appropriateness, correctness, completeness, and usefulness of the material on these pages.

Since the author is not a licensed medical practitioner, the material in this book shouldn't be interpreted as medical advice. Before making any modifications to their diet, exercise regimen, or medical treatment, readers are urged to speak with a licensed healthcare provider.

Moreover, the author has no connection to any of the businesses, organizations, or people that are discussed in this book. Any mentions of goods, services, businesses, or people are purely informative and do not indicate endorsement or suggestion.

This book's content is entirely dependent on the author's expertise, study, and comprehension of the topic. Despite having taken reasonable care to offer correct information, the author disclaims all liability for any mistakes or omissions in the material as well as for any losses, harm, or damages resulting from using the information.

It is recommended that readers use their own judgment and discretion when applying the knowledge in this book to their own situations. The use or implementation of any material in this book may result in unfavorable repercussions, directly or indirectly, for which the author assumes no liability.

By reading this book, you agree to release and hold the author harmless from any claims, losses, liabilities, costs, or expenditures resulting from or related to the use of the information you get from it.

Table of Contents

ABOUT THIS BOOK

"Cholecystitis: A Comprehensive Guide to Understanding and Managing Gallbladder Inflammation" is an invaluable resource for anybody looking to learn more about this common medical issue. From the minute you open its pages, you'll be taken on a voyage of enlightenment and empowerment, learning insights that might save lives.

Chapter 1 provides the groundwork by exposing the reader to the complexities of cholecystitis, uncovering its secrets, and offering a comprehensive knowledge of the gallbladder's involvement in the disease. Understanding the core causes and risk factors, as discussed in Chapter 2, allows readers to identify warning signals early on, possibly avoiding major repercussions.

What distinguishes this book is its focus on empowerment via knowledge. Chapter 3 digs into diagnostic tools, enabling readers to better communicate with their healthcare professionals, resulting in accurate and prompt diagnoses. With this information, readers may safely choose the treatment choices presented in Chapter 4, whether they prefer conservative measures or surgical surgery.

Furthermore, the book expands its scope beyond medical procedures. The lifestyle changes discussed in Chapter 5 provide comprehensive methods for controlling cholecystitis, stressing the relevance of dietary changes, exercise, and stress management. Post-treatment care, as detailed in Chapter 6, offers vital assistance for recovery and long-term maintenance, assuring a seamless return to health.

Chapter 7 faces the unpleasant reality of consequences, informing readers about the dangers of untreated cholecystitis and providing preventative options. Meanwhile, Chapter 8 offers realistic dietary advice to help patients navigate their nutritional demands.

Perhaps the most engaging component of this book is Chapter 9, which features patient viewpoints and real-life tales of resistance and victory. Readers may receive sympathy, inspiration, and practical counsel from individuals who have been through similar experiences.

Chapter 10 provides a view into the future, highlighting advances in cholecystitis research and new therapies, instilling hope and optimism in both patients and healthcare professionals.

"Cholecystitis" is more than simply a book; it is a lifeline for everyone affected by this ailment. Its thorough approach, intelligent advice, and motivating stories make it an essential companion on the path to health and well-being.

CHAPTER 1

What Is Cholecystitis?

Cholecystitis is a disorder caused by inflammation of the gallbladder, a tiny organ found under the liver. The gallbladder mainly stores bile, which is a digestive fluid generated by the liver. When bile is required for digestion, the gallbladder contracts and empties into the small intestine. Cholecystitis develops when the bile ducts leading to the gallbladder get clogged, usually by gallstones, causing bile to collect and the gallbladder to become inflamed.

Understanding The Gallbladder

To truly appreciate cholecystitis, one must first understand the gallbladder's function in digestion. The gallbladder serves as a bile storage reservoir, which is necessary for the breakdown of lipids in our diet. When we eat a fatty meal, our gallbladder contracts and releases bile into the small intestine via the bile ducts. The bile emulsifies lipids, making them simpler to digest and absorb. Without a properly functioning gallbladder, this process may be disturbed, resulting in digestive problems and pain.

Causes And Risk Factors

Several variables may influence the development of cholecystitis. The most frequent cause is gallstones, which are hardened deposits of digestive fluid that may develop in the gallbladder. When gallstones obstruct the bile ducts or the cystic duct (the tube that connects the gallbladder to the bile duct), bile cannot flow normally, causing inflammation and irritation to the gallbladder walls.

Other risk factors for cholecystitis are:

1. Obesity: Excess body weight increases the likelihood of developing gallstones, which may lead

to cholecystitis. Obesity is often connected with poor eating habits, which may lead to gallstone development.

2. **Gender and Age:** Women are more likely than males to develop gallstones, particularly if they are pregnant or receiving hormone replacement treatment. Additionally, cholecystitis is more prevalent in those over the age of 40.

3. Crash diets or quick weight reduction programs may increase the chance of getting gallstones because the liver releases additional cholesterol into bile during rapid weight loss, contributing to stone formation.

4. **Diabetes:** People with diabetes are more likely to develop gallstones, which may be linked to changes in bile composition.

5. Genetics: Family history may influence the development of cholecystitis. If you have close relatives who have had gallstones or cholecystitis, you may be more at risk.

Understanding the causes and risk factors is critical for avoiding and treating cholecystitis. Individuals may lower their chance of acquiring this unpleasant illness by dealing with underlying concerns such as obesity, a poor diet, and quick weight reduction. Early identification and treatment of gallstones might also assist in avoiding complications like cholecystitis.

CHAPTER 2

Signs And Symptoms

Recognizing The Warning Signs

Recognizing the warning symptoms of cholecystitis is critical for timely diagnosis and treatment. Symptoms of cholecystitis usually appear when the gallbladder is inflamed or blocked. One of the most common symptoms is severe stomach discomfort, which is frequently localized in the upper right quadrant. The discomfort may be intense and may spread to the back or shoulder blades. It usually happens after eating a fatty meal and might last for hours.

Along with the discomfort, people may have nausea and vomiting, particularly if the inflammation is severe. Some people may notice a yellowing of the skin and whites of their eyes, which is known as jaundice. This happens when bile flow is impeded, resulting in bilirubin accumulation in the circulation. Additionally, fever and chills may appear, suggesting a gallbladder infection.

It is critical to pay attention to these warning symptoms, particularly if they continue or worsen with time. Ignoring them may result in problems such as gallbladder rupture, which is potentially fatal. Seeking medical care right once is critical for accurate diagnosis and treatment.

Differentiating Acute And Chronic Cholecystitis

Cholecystitis may be acute or chronic, with each having specific features.

Acute cholecystitis is characterized by fast onset and severe symptoms. Abdominal discomfort is usually severe and continuous, with fever and chills. Patients may suffer nausea, vomiting, and jaundice. Acute cholecystitis is mainly caused by gallstones obstructing the cystic duct, resulting in gallbladder inflammation and infection. Prompt medical attention is required to relieve symptoms and avoid consequences.

Chronic cholecystitis, on the other hand, progresses slowly over time. Patients may have recurring bouts of minor stomach discomfort, particularly after eating fatty meals. Other symptoms may include bloating, gas, and indigestion. Chronic cholecystitis is often linked with gallstones, however it may also develop in the absence of them. While the symptoms may be less severe than those of acute cholecystitis, they may nevertheless influence the individual's quality of life. Long-term treatment options may include dietary modifications and medication to alleviate symptoms.

When To Seek Medical Attention

Knowing when to seek medical help for cholecystitis is critical for prompt treatment and avoidance of consequences. If you encounter any of the following symptoms, you should visit a healthcare professional:

• Prolonged stomach discomfort, particularly in the upper right quadrant.

• Fever and chills might suggest an infection.

• Symptoms may include nausea, vomiting, and jaundice.

• Yellowing of skin and whites of eyes.

• Symptoms of a serious problem, such as gallbladder rupture, include difficulty breathing and fast pulse.

If you have a history of gallstones or cholecystitis, you must be attentive to any changes in symptoms. Even if the symptoms seem moderate at first, they may quickly worsen, especially in acute cholecystitis. Seeking medical assistance as soon as possible will help avoid problems and ensure that you receive the proper treatment.

CHAPTER 3

Diagnostic Tools

Exploring Diagnostic Tests

Healthcare practitioners use a range of diagnostic tests to help them diagnose cholecystitis. Ultrasound imaging is a fundamental weapon in their arsenal. This non-invasive treatment lets physicians look into the abdomen, notably the gallbladder area, for symptoms of inflammation or gallstones. Ultrasound is preferred for its efficacy, safety, and cost-effectiveness, making it a popular choice in many medical contexts.

In addition to ultrasonography, blood tests are important in detecting cholecystitis. These tests, such as liver function tests and white blood cell counts, may provide important information about the gallbladder's function and the presence of infection or inflammation.

Elevations in specific liver enzymes or white blood cell counts might be cause for concern, prompting additional inquiry into cholecystitis.

In addition, diagnostic methods may involve a physical examination to evaluate the patient's symptoms and general health. Clinicians pay particular attention to certain symptoms, such as abdominal discomfort, fever, and jaundice, which might indicate gallbladder problems.

Role Of Imaging Techniques

While ultrasound remains the primary diagnostic tool for cholecystitis, newer imaging modalities such as CT scans and MRI scans provide extra clarity in difficult situations. Computed Tomography (CT) scans use a sequence of X-ray pictures collected from various angles to produce comprehensive cross-sectional images of the body. This lets healthcare workers see the gallbladder and surrounding tissues with more accuracy, assisting in the detection of problems such as abscesses or perforation.

Magnetic resonance imaging (MRI) is another excellent diagnostic technique. MRI uses magnetic fields and radio waves to create high-resolution pictures of the body without the need for ionizing radiation. This makes it especially effective for examining soft tissues and finding abnormalities in the gallbladder or bile ducts. MRI may offer vital information regarding the degree of inflammation and any related consequences, allowing for more effective treatment options.

The Value Of Accurate Diagnosis

In the case of cholecystitis, a correct diagnosis is critical for commencing prompt and suitable therapy. Misdiagnosis or delayed diagnosis might result in increased symptoms, complications, or even surgical crises. Healthcare practitioners may confidently identify the underlying cause of symptoms using a mix of diagnostic tests and imaging modalities.

A precise diagnosis not only relieves the patient's pain but also assures the best possible results by adapting treatment strategies to each individual's requirements. Whether it is cautious antibiotic treatment or surgical removal of the gallbladder, a clear diagnosis is the cornerstone for successful therapy.

Furthermore, correct diagnosis allows healthcare practitioners to track the course of therapy and detect any possible consequences early. Regular follow-up examinations and imaging investigations allow for continuous monitoring of the patient's state, ensuring that therapies are changed as necessary to promote healing and avoid recurrence.

Finally, the diagnosis of cholecystitis requires a multifaceted approach that includes a variety of assays and imaging modalities. Each tool serves a distinct function in unraveling the nuances of the ailment, eventually paving the way for the best patient treatment and results.

CHAPTER 4

Treatment Options

Conservative Approaches (Dietary Changes, Medications)

Conservative treatments are critical in controlling cholecystitis, particularly in moderate instances or when surgery is not urgently required. One of the most important methods is to change your nutrition. Patients are often recommended to have a low-fat diet, since high-fat meals may cause gallbladder spasms, resulting in discomfort and inflammation. Emphasizing nutritious grains, fruits, vegetables, and lean meats while limiting saturated and trans fats will assist with symptoms.

Furthermore, drugs may be provided to relieve the discomfort and inflammation caused by cholecystitis. Nonsteroidal anti-inflammatory medicines (NSAIDs), such as ibuprofen or acetaminophen, may help relieve discomfort. Antibiotics may also be recommended if there is an indication of infection. These drugs assist to combat the bacterial infection that may occasionally accompany cholecystitis.

Furthermore, lifestyle changes are often suggested to lessen the likelihood of recurring episodes. Maintaining a healthy weight via food and exercise helps reduce the chance of gallstone development, a major cause of cholecystitis. Avoiding fast weight loss and crash diets may help prevent gallstones from developing.

Patients are typically recommended to remain hydrated and drink plenty of fluids every day. This helps maintain bile moving freely and prevents it from getting excessively concentrated, lowering the chance of gallstones. Regular physical exercise may also improve digestion and lower the risk of gallstones.

To summarize, conservative methods of cholecystitis treatment include dietary adjustments, symptom-management drugs, and lifestyle changes to avoid recurrence. Patients who use these measures may typically successfully control their disease and enhance their overall health.

Surgical Intervention (Cholecystectomy)

When conservative treatments fail to offer relief or problems emerge, surgical intervention, often a cholecystectomy, may be required. A cholecystectomy is the surgical removal of the gallbladder and is considered the last therapy for cholecystitis, especially in situations of acute or recurring infection.

There are two basic methods for doing a cholecystectomy: laparoscopic and open surgery. The recommended approach is laparoscopic cholecystectomy, which is less intrusive and has a shorter recovery period. This treatment involves making small incisions in the belly and inserting a tiny camera (laparoscope) and surgical equipment to remove the gallbladder.

In contrast, an open cholecystectomy requires a bigger incision in the belly to directly reach and remove the gallbladder. This method may be required in specific situations, such as when there are problems or the surgeon faces difficulty performing a laparoscopic treatment.

Most patients may resume regular activities within a few days to a week after having a cholecystectomy, depending on the kind of surgery and their specific recovery time. However, it is critical to carefully follow post-operative instructions, including dietary advice and activity limitations, to guarantee adequate healing and reduce the chance of problems.

While a cholecystectomy completely removes the danger of recurring cholecystitis and gallstones, it's crucial to remember that the gallbladder is not an essential organ, and its removal seldom causes substantial long-term health issues. Most individuals can have a regular, healthy life without their gallbladder.

In conclusion, surgical intervention, especially cholecystectomy, is a very successful therapeutic option for cholecystitis, providing long-term symptom alleviation while lowering the risk of complications.

Emerging Therapies And Alternative Medicine

In addition to traditional treatments, various developing therapies and alternative medicine techniques show promise in the management of cholecystitis, either as supplementary treatments or as non-surgical alternatives.

One promising treatment gaining traction is oral dissolution therapy, which entails gently dissolving gallstones using medicines. This method is most helpful for people with tiny, cholesterol-based stones and may take many months to provide effects. While not appropriate in all situations, it may be a non-invasive alternative to surgery for certain people.

Another new area of study is gallbladder stenting. In this treatment, a stent is put into the bile duct to relieve blockage and improve bile flow, which may help reduce cholecystitis symptoms, especially in individuals who are not surgical candidates or need temporary relief before surgery.

Patients looking for natural therapies for cholecystitis may also consider alternative medical methods such as acupuncture, herbal supplements, and nutritional supplements. While there is minimal scientific evidence to support the usefulness of these techniques, some people experience symptom alleviation and enhanced well-being after using them. Patients must consult with their healthcare physician before pursuing any alternative treatments to confirm their safety and compatibility with their entire treatment plan.

New therapies and alternative medicine provide additional possibilities for treating cholecystitis, either as supplements to traditional treatments or as alternatives for people who choose non-surgical procedures. More study is required to completely understand the efficacy and safety of these therapies, although they show promise in terms of improving outcomes and quality of life for cholecystitis patients.

CHAPTER 5

Lifestyle Modifications

Dietary Recommendations For Cholecystitis

When it comes to controlling cholecystitis with dietary changes, it's important to understand how specific foods affect your gallbladder health. One of the key aims is to lessen the stress on your gallbladder, which entails avoiding meals heavy in fat and cholesterol. These may cause unpleasant sensations by stimulating your gallbladder to contract more often.

Instead, concentrate on adding more fiber-rich foods to your diet. Fiber aids digestion by encouraging regular bowel movements and reducing constipation, which may worsen cholecystitis symptoms. Choose whole grains, fruits, veggies, and legumes to enhance your fiber intake.

Furthermore, it is critical to keep hydrated. Drinking enough water supports bile production and keeps your digestive system running normally. Aim for at least eight glasses of water every day, and try adding lemon juice to your water to increase bile movement.

In addition to fiber and water, try including meals high in antioxidants and anti-inflammatory compounds. These may help minimize gallbladder inflammation and pain. Berries, leafy greens, salmon, and olive oil are among examples.

Finally, portion management is important for controlling cholecystitis symptoms. Eating smaller, more frequent meals throughout the day will reduce the strain on your gallbladder and prevent it from being overloaded with food at once. Avoiding big, heavy meals may help lessen the chance of unpleasant bouts.

Exercise And Physical Activity

Regular exercise is an important part of a healthy lifestyle, particularly for those who have cholecystitis. Physical exercise may benefit you in a variety of ways, including weight control and improved digestion.

Cardiovascular workouts like brisk walking, running, cycling, or swimming are especially good for those who have cholecystitis. These exercises enhance blood flow throughout the body, including the digestive organs, which aids in the effective digestion of bile and other digestive fluids.

Strength training routines may also aid in maintaining muscle mass and improve overall metabolism. However, exercises that exert too much tension on the abdominal muscles, such as heavy lifting or hardcore workouts, should be avoided since they might worsen cholecystitis symptoms.

Exercise requires a high level of consistency. Aim for at least 30 minutes of moderate-intensity exercise on most days of the week. If you are new to exercising or have worries about your fitness level, engage with a healthcare expert or a licensed personal trainer to create a safe and efficient workout regimen that is suited to your specific requirements.

Incorporating physical exercise into your routine may also help you manage stress, which leads us to the following topic.

Stress Management Techniques

Stress may have a substantial influence on digestive health, such as worsening cholecystitis symptoms. As a result, persons suffering from this ailment must use stress management measures.

Deep breathing exercises are an efficient stress-management method. Taking slow, deep breaths activates the body's relaxation response, which aids in stress reduction and promotes a sensation of peace. Deep breathing exercises should be done for a few minutes every day, particularly when you're stressed or anxious.

Another useful approach is mindfulness meditation. Mindfulness is the practice of paying attention to the present moment without judgment, which may help reduce stress and promote emotional well-being. Consider introducing brief mindfulness meditation sessions into your daily routine to assist manage cholecystitis-related stress.

Additionally, participating in activities that you love and find calming might help to reduce stress. Make time for things that offer you pleasure and help you decompress, such as reading, listening to music, going for a walk outside, or practicing hobbies.

It is also critical to emphasize sleep hygiene, since insufficient sleep may raise stress and aggravate cholecystitis symptoms. Aim for seven to nine hours of excellent sleep every night by sticking to a consistent sleep schedule, maintaining a pleasant sleep environment, and practicing relaxation methods before bedtime.

Individuals with cholecystitis may better manage their disease and enhance their overall quality of life by integrating lifestyle modifications such as dietary changes, frequent exercise, and stress management strategies.

CHAPTER 6

Post-Treatment Care

Recovery Process After Surgery

The healing process for cholecystitis starts after surgery, whether laparoscopic or open. During the first recuperation phase, which usually lasts a few days, patients are carefully followed in the hospital to ensure that no problems arise. Pain management is an important part of post-operative treatment, and patients are often given pain medicines to relieve discomfort.

Patients often report discomfort, edema, and bruising around the incision sites. This is very normal and generally passes within a few days. To speed up the healing process and limit the risk of infection, keep the incision sites clean and dry.

Following surgery, patients may be recommended to gradually resume solid meals in their diet. To reduce stress on the digestive tract, start with a bland and low-fat diet. To avoid difficulties, follow any dietary instructions recommended by healthcare providers.

Light physical exercise, such as brief walks, may assist to improve circulation and avoid blood clots. However, it is critical to avoid overexertion and to heed the body's warnings. Rest are equally important part of the rehabilitation process.

As the days pass, patients should progressively feel stronger and more like themselves. However, it is critical to follow any post-operative recommendations given by the surgical team, such as limitations on moving heavy things and driving.

During the recuperation time, it is natural to feel a variety of feelings such as relief, worry, and dissatisfaction. It might be beneficial to rely on friends and family for support at this time, as well as to talk honestly with healthcare practitioners about any worries or queries.

In certain circumstances, rehabilitation or physical therapy may be suggested to help with recovery, especially if the patient has problems or underlying health conditions before surgery. Overall, patience, self-care, and following physician recommendations are essential components of a successful recovery after cholecystitis surgery.

Follow-Up Visits And Monitoring

Following cholecystitis surgery, frequent follow-up appointments with healthcare specialists are required to monitor the healing process and guarantee the best possible recovery. These visits often take place in the weeks and months after surgery, allowing healthcare specialists to check the patient's development and handle any issues or difficulties that may emerge.

During follow-up visits, healthcare practitioners may do physical exams, examine laboratory test findings, and conduct imaging scans to assess the gallbladder and surrounding tissues. This thorough approach ensures that any concerns are discovered and handled as soon as possible.

In addition to monitoring the physical components of healing, follow-up sessions allow patients to address any remaining symptoms or concerns they may have. This open communication between patients and healthcare professionals is critical to ensure that patients feel supported and informed throughout their rehabilitation.

Follow-up appointments may be planned more or less often depending on the patient's specific needs. Patients who have a history of cholecystitis or other gallbladder problems may need more regular monitoring to avoid recurrence or consequences.

In addition to follow-up visits with healthcare experts, patients may be urged to undertake lifestyle changes to improve general health and avoid recurrent bouts of cholecystitis. This may involve dietary modifications, such as cutting down on fatty or fried meals, as well as increasing physical exercise and maintaining a healthy weight.

Overall, cholecystitis post-treatment care must include frequent follow-up visits and monitoring. Patients who remain involved in their treatment and follow medical recommendations may assist in guaranteeing a smooth and successful recovery.

Coping Strategies For Long-Term Management

Living with cholecystitis, whether treated by medication, lifestyle modifications, or surgery, may be difficult for people. However, various coping tactics may help people manage their health and enhance their quality of life in the long run.

One important coping mechanism is education. Understanding the underlying causes of cholecystitis, as well as the treatment choices available, may help patients take an active part in their care. Healthcare practitioners may give patients useful information and tools to help them better understand their condition and make educated choices about their treatment.

Self-care is another effective coping approach. This involves developing healthy lifestyle habits including eating a well-balanced diet, exercising frequently, getting adequate sleep, and managing stress. These lifestyle adjustments may help lessen the frequency and severity of cholecystitis flare-ups while also improving overall health.

Dealing with cholecystitis requires support from friends, family, and healthcare professionals. A robust support network may provide emotional support, practical aid, and encouragement during challenging times. Individuals suffering from cholecystitis might benefit greatly from support groups and internet forums.

In addition to these techniques, people should openly talk with their healthcare professionals about any symptoms or concerns they may have. Regular check-ups and monitoring may help detect problems early on and avoid consequences.

Finally, having a good attitude and being resilient in the face of adversity is critical for long-term cholecystitis therapy. Living with a chronic disease may be difficult, but taking a proactive approach to self-care and getting assistance when required can help people manage their symptoms and live full lives.

CHAPTER 7

Complications

Potential Risks Of Untreated Cholecystitis

Untreated cholecystitis may cause a variety of consequences, including life-threatening conditions. When gallstones block the cystic duct, bile accumulates, creating an environment conducive to infection. If left untreated, this inflammation may expand beyond the gallbladder, resulting in a variety of problems. One such danger is the establishment of an abscess in the gallbladder, which may burst and cause peritonitis, a serious abdominal infection. Furthermore, untreated cholecystitis increases the danger of developing gangrene inside the gallbladder and needing emergency surgery.

Furthermore, chronic inflammation may cause the production of adhesions, and fibrous bands that bind organs together. These adhesions may cause intestinal blockage, resulting in severe stomach discomfort, bloating, and vomiting. Furthermore, untreated cholecystitis may cause choledocholithiasis, a disorder in which gallstones move from the gallbladder to the common bile duct. This blockage may block the passage of bile into the intestines, resulting in jaundice, severe stomach discomfort, and pancreatitis.

Secondary Complications And Their Management

Secondary problems might develop as a result of untreated cholecystitis, demanding careful treatment to avoid serious consequences. One such consequence is cholangitis, which is an inflammation of the bile ducts. This illness produces symptoms such as fever, jaundice, and stomach discomfort. To reduce the spread of infection and avoid septicemia, broad-spectrum antibiotics should be administered as soon as possible, followed by biliary drainage.

Furthermore, persistent gallstones may cause bile duct strictures, which constrict the route for bile flow. Endoscopic retrograde cholangiopancreatography (ERCP) combined with stent implantation or balloon dilatation is the foundation for treating these strictures, restoring bile flow, and relieving associated symptoms. Furthermore, if gallstones enter the pancreatic duct, severe pancreatitis may develop, demanding urgent supportive treatment and pain management while treating the underlying cause.

Strategies For Prevention

The key to avoiding cholecystitis and its sequelae is prevention. Dietary changes are critical in reducing gallstone development, with a focus on eating a diet high in fiber, low in saturated fats, and high in fruits and vegetables. Furthermore, keeping a healthy weight and avoiding fast weight reduction will help reduce the chance of gallstone development.

Regular physical activity, for example, helps to promote bile flow and reduce stasis, which improves gallbladder health. Furthermore, quitting smoking and limiting alcohol use may help minimize the incidence of gallstone development and subsequent cholecystitis. Individuals at high risk, such as those with a family history of gallstones or certain medical problems, need proactive screening and early management to avoid cholecystitis and its repercussions.

Identifying the possible hazards of untreated cholecystitis, treating subsequent complications cautiously, and implementing preventative actions are critical in protecting against the negative impacts of this illness. Individuals may reduce their risk of cholecystitis and maintain gallbladder health by taking proactive steps and intervening when necessary, boosting overall well-being and quality of life.

CHAPTER 8

Dietary Guidelines

Foods To Avoid

To manage cholecystitis, it is critical to understand which foods might worsen symptoms and even cause painful bouts. While everyone's tolerance for certain meals varies, there are a few typical offenders to avoid.

1. **rich-Fat Foods:** Foods rich in saturated and trans fats may cause pain for those with cholecystitis because they encourage the gallbladder to constrict. This includes fried meals, fatty meats, processed snacks such as chips and pastries, and creamy sauces.

2. Spicy meals may irritate the digestive system, perhaps causing gallbladder inflammation. Avoid

dishes that include spicy peppers, chili powder, or an overabundance of garlic and onions.

3. Dairy Products: Some persons with cholecystitis struggle to digest full-fat dairy products such as whole milk, cheese, and cream. Low-fat or dairy-free options may be preferable.

4. High-Fiber Foods: While fiber is typically useful for digestion, excessive amounts may produce gas, bloating, and pain in those with cholecystitis. Foods rich in insoluble fiber, such as whole grains and raw vegetables, may need to be avoided.

5. Alcohol and caffeine both stimulate the gallbladder and digestive tract, which may lead to cholecystitis symptoms. These drinks should be consumed in moderation or avoided completely.

6. Carbonated Beverages: The carbonation in sodas and fizzy beverages may cause bloating and discomfort, especially in those with sensitive stomachs or cholecystitis.

7. Processed meals often include chemicals, preservatives, and harmful fats, which may exacerbate inflammation and digestive problems. Choosing entire, unprocessed meals is often a superior option.

Recommended Dietary Modifications

Dietary changes may help relieve symptoms and avoid flare-ups of cholecystitis. Here are some suggested adjustments to consider:

1. **Focus on Whole Foods:** Eat a diet high in whole grains, lean meats, fruits, and vegetables. These meals are simpler to digest and less likely to cause symptoms.

2. **Choose Lean Proteins:** Instead of fatty meats, choose lean protein sources including chicken, fish,

tofu, and lentils. These proteins are lower in fat and so less prone to trigger the gallbladder.

3. Incorporate Healthy Fats: While high-fat meals should be avoided, small quantities of healthy fats like avocados, nuts, seeds, and olive oil may supply important nutrients without causing symptoms.

4. Stay Hydrated: Drinking lots of water is essential for good overall health and digestion. Aim for at least eight glasses of water each day, and flavor with lemon or cucumber to avoid adding calories or sugar.

5. Eat Smaller, More Frequent Meals: Rather than huge meals, choose smaller, more frequent meals throughout the day. This may assist to avoid overloading the digestive system and reduce the likelihood of triggering symptoms.

6. Keep track of portion sizes, particularly when it comes to high-fat or rich meals. Eating in smaller quantities may help avoid overeating and discomfort.

Sample Meal Plans For Cholecystitis Patients

Creating balanced meal planning may help people with cholecystitis manage their symptoms and stay healthy. Here are some example meal options to consider:

Breakfast:

• Top your oatmeal with fresh fruit and almonds.

• Enjoy whole grain toast with avocado and tomato.

• Greek yogurt parfait with honey and almonds.

Lunch:

• Grilled chicken salad served with mixed greens, cherry tomatoes, and balsamic vinaigrette.

• Quinoa salad with cucumber, bell peppers, feta, and lemon-tahini dressing.

• Serve lentil soup with whole-grain toast.

Dinner:

• Baked salmon served with roasted sweet potatoes and broccoli.

• Stir-fried tofu, mixed veggies, and brown rice

• Turkey meatballs with marinara sauce served over zucchini noodles.

Snacks:

• Apple slices with almond butter.

• Hummus with carrot sticks.

• Greek yogurt and granola

Individuals suffering from cholecystitis may enhance their overall quality of life by adhering to this dietary advice and eating balanced meals. It's critical to collaborate with a healthcare professional or registered dietitian to create a meal plan that suits your specific requirements and interests.

CHAPTER 9

Patient Perspectives

Tips From Survivors And Thrivers

Navigating the obstacles of cholecystitis may be difficult, but hearing from individuals who have successfully conquered them can give essential insights. Survivors and thrivers of cholecystitis often have personal experience of what works and what does not when it comes to treating the ailment. Their counsel might vary from practical lifestyle modifications to emotional support measures that can make a big impact on one's rehabilitation.

Dietary And Lifestyle Changes

One typical piece of advice from survivors is to pay special attention to your eating habits. Certain foods might cause cholecystitis symptoms, thus dietary changes are typically necessary.

Many people find success by eating a low-fat diet, avoiding greasy or fried foods, and eating smaller, more often meals to reduce the strain on the gallbladder. Fiber-rich meals, including fruits, vegetables, and whole grains, may help improve digestive health and lower the likelihood of flare-ups.

Lifestyle adjustments, in addition to food changes, may be very important in controlling cholecystitis. Regular exercise, for example, may help you maintain a healthy weight and feel better overall. Stress management practices, such as meditation or yoga, may also be useful since stress may worsen symptoms for some people. By proactively addressing lifestyle variables, cholecystitis survivors may improve their condition and quality of life.

Medication Management And Follow-Up Care

Another helpful recommendation from survivors is to be proactive with medication management and follow-up treatment. Depending on the severity of the problem, healthcare experts may prescribe drugs to treat symptoms or avoid further consequences. It is important to take prescription drugs as instructed and to disclose any concerns or adverse effects to your healthcare staff.

Furthermore, frequent follow-up meetings are essential for tracking improvement and managing changes in symptoms or health status. Survivors underline the necessity of being educated about their health and actively engaging in their treatment plan. This preventive strategy may assist in avoiding cholecystitis recurrence and assure good long-term care.

Overcoming Challenges And Staying Positive

While cholecystitis brings various hurdles, adopting a cheerful attitude may make a significant difference in dealing with the disease. Survivors and thrivers often discuss ideas for overcoming challenges and being resilient in the face of adversity.

Seeking And Building A Support Network

One of the most effective techniques for overcoming obstacles is to seek assistance from individuals who understand what you're going through. Sharing experiences and resources, whether via internet connections or participation in local support groups, may provide comfort and encouragement. Many survivors take comfort in knowing they are not alone on their path, and they draw strength from the collective knowledge of their peers.

Creating a support network of friends, family members, and healthcare professionals is also critical. These people can provide practical help, emotional support, and encouragement during tough times. By surrounding yourself with a supportive environment, you may better negotiate the obstacles of cholecystitis and retain a good attitude.

Embracing Self-Care And Prioritizing Well-Being.

It's easy to forget about self-care when dealing with cholecystitis, but maintaining your health is critical for resilience and recovery. Survivors underline the significance of listening to your body, practicing self-compassion, and establishing boundaries as needed. Taking time for things that provide pleasure and relaxation might assist in reducing stress and improve overall health.

Self-care is more than just physical health; it also includes mental and emotional well-being. Hobbies, mindfulness practice, and professional counseling or therapy may all help you maintain a happy attitude and enhance your quality of life. By engaging in self-care activities, cholecystitis survivors may build resilience and flourish despite the obstacles they experience.

In conclusion, cholecystitis survivors and thrivers provide vital advice about managing the ailment and keeping a good mindset. Individuals may improve their symptoms and avoid recurrence by implementing dietary modifications, lifestyle changes, and proactive healthcare management into their daily routine. Overcoming obstacles requires getting help, practicing self-care, and prioritizing well-being, but with persistence and tenacity, it is possible to flourish in the face of adversity.

CHAPTER 10

Future Directions

Advancements In Cholecystitis Research

Cholecystitis research has advanced at a rapid rate in recent years, owing to advances in medical technology and a better knowledge of the disease's underlying causes. Diagnostic procedures are one area that has seen substantial development. Ultrasound and CT scans are traditional approaches, however novel imaging modalities such as magnetic resonance cholangiopancreatography (MRCP) and endoscopic ultrasound (EUS) have been introduced. These approaches provide increased resolution and accuracy in identifying gallbladder inflammation, allowing for earlier diagnosis and treatment planning.

Another fascinating prospect in cholecystitis research is the discovery of biomarkers.

Researchers are constantly exploring numerous biomolecules, such as proteins and genetic markers, that may serve as biomarkers of gallbladder inflammation. The discovery of accurate biomarkers might transform cholecystitis diagnosis, enabling faster and more precise detection of the ailment.

Furthermore, there has been a rise in studies into the microbiome's function in cholecystitis. Studies have found a complicated relationship between gut bacteria and gallbladder health, with dysbiosis possibly leading to inflammation. Understanding these microbial dynamics may lead to new treatment options, such as probiotics or fecal microbiota transplantation, for restoring microbial balance and alleviating cholecystitis symptoms.

In addition to diagnostic and therapeutic advances, researchers are investigating the genetic basis of cholecystitis. Genome-wide association studies (GWAS) have found genetic changes linked to an increased risk of gallbladder disease, providing insight into the hereditary components that underpin the disorder. This insight might pave the way for customized medical techniques, in which medicines are matched to an individual's genetic profile for maximum effectiveness.

As cholecystitis research advances, multidisciplinary cooperation and the use of cutting-edge technology will be critical drivers of development. By utilizing these breakthroughs, healthcare practitioners may improve patient treatment and outcomes, eventually enhancing the quality of life for those living with this prevalent but potentially catastrophic disorder.

Promising Treatments On The Horizon

The therapy landscape for cholecystitis is changing dramatically, with potential medicines on the horizon that give patients fresh hope.

One such advancement is the introduction of less invasive techniques for gallstone removal. While surgical cholecystectomy has long been the gold standard therapy for symptomatic gallstones, advances in endoscopic technology have made it possible to remove stones from the gallbladder and bile ducts without requiring open surgery. Endoscopic retrograde cholangiopancreatography (ERCP) and laparoscopic cholecystectomy are increasingly common procedures, with faster recovery periods and a lower risk of complications than older surgical techniques.

Another promising area of research is the development of pharmacological treatments for cholecystitis. Traditional treatment methods have centered on symptom management and complication prevention, often including the use of pain relievers and antibiotics. However, researchers are currently looking at new pharmacological targets and therapeutic compounds that might modulate the inflammatory response and improve gallbladder function. These developing medicines, which range from anti-inflammatory drugs to gallstone-dissolving pharmaceuticals, have the potential to change cholecystitis therapy by providing more effective and customized solutions to patients.

Furthermore, regenerative medicine shows promise in repairing and rebuilding damaged gallbladder tissue. Preclinical research using stem cells and tissue engineering approaches has shown promising results in boosting tissue healing and restoring normal function in animal models of cholecystitis. While clinical trials are still in their early phases, the promise of regenerative therapeutics provides a tantalizing view into the future of cholecystitis therapy, in which damaged organs may be restored rather than just maintained.

In addition to these treatment advances, lifestyle changes and nutritional interventions are critical in cholecystitis therapy. Patients are being advised to develop good eating habits, such as a well-balanced diet rich in fruits, vegetables, and fiber, and to avoid eating too many fatty and fried meals. Furthermore, regular exercise and weight control are recommended to lower the chance of gallstone development and improve cholecystitis symptoms.

As research advances and new medicines become available, the future for cholecystitis patients is bright. By embracing these technologies and taking a complete approach to care, healthcare practitioners may give patients individualized treatment plans suited to their specific requirements, eventually enhancing outcomes and quality of life.

Empowering Patients Through Education And Advocacy

Empowering patients with information and support is critical in the care of cholecystitis, allowing them to make educated health choices and successfully advocate for their own needs. Education is essential in this process since patients must understand the nature of their ailment, including its origins, symptoms, and treatment alternatives. Healthcare practitioners play an important role in patient education by giving clear and accurate information that is easy to comprehend and acquire.

Furthermore, patient advocacy organizations and support networks play an important role in empowering people with cholecystitis. These groups allow patients to connect with others who are experiencing similar issues, share their stories, and have access to resources and support. Patient advocacy organizations assist people manage their healthcare journeys with confidence and resilience by instilling a feeling of community and togetherness.

Furthermore, patient empowerment involves more than just information and assistance; it also includes active engagement in healthcare decision-making. Patients are encouraged to ask questions, express concerns, and work with their healthcare professionals to create tailored treatment plans that reflect their choices and objectives. Shared decision-making encourages patient autonomy and ensures that treatment techniques are customized to individual requirements, resulting in better results and more patient satisfaction with care.

In addition to individual empowerment, advocating at the societal level is critical for promoting legislative changes and increasing awareness of cholecystitis and other illnesses. Patients and advocacy organizations may effect substantial change and improve outcomes for people suffering from cholecystitis by campaigning for more research funding, better access to healthcare services, and enhanced public knowledge.

Overall, by empowering patients via information, support, and advocacy, we can create a healthcare system that emphasizes patient-centered treatment and promotes favorable outcomes for people with cholecystitis. Through cooperation and collective action, we can build a future in which every patient gets the information, resources, and support they need to properly manage their disease and live their best lives.

CONCLUSION

To summarize, cholecystitis is a dangerous inflammatory illness of the gallbladder that needs immediate medical attention and adequate treatment to avoid consequences. This illness is often caused by gallstones blocking the cystic duct, resulting in bile buildup and inflammation of the gallbladder wall.

Cholecystitis is often characterized by severe stomach discomfort, fever, nausea, vomiting, and soreness in the upper right quadrant of the abdomen. Prompt diagnosis is critical, and imaging investigations like ultrasound or computed tomography (CT) scans can confirm the diagnosis and determine the severity of the problem.

Treatment options for cholecystitis differ based on the severity of the symptoms and the patient's general condition. In mild instances, conservative treatment with fasting, intravenous fluids, and antibiotics may be enough to relieve symptoms and avoid problems. However, in more severe instances or those with consequences such as gangrene or gallbladder perforation, surgical intervention, usually a laparoscopic cholecystectomy, is sometimes required to remove the gallbladder and relieve symptoms.

Postoperative care is vital for a smooth recovery and reducing the risk of complications. Patients should be continuously followed for evidence of infection or other surgical problems, and appropriate pain treatment and dietary changes should be undertaken to speed up recovery and avoid recurrence.

In conclusion, although cholecystitis may be a painful and possibly fatal illness, prompt diagnosis and treatment can lead to positive results for individuals. Close coordination among patients, healthcare professionals, and surgeons is required to guarantee the best treatment and results for those impacted by this disorder.

THE END

9 798325 370472